LICENSED TO KILL

THE GROWING EPIDEMICS OF IATROGENIC DISEASE AND BUREAUCRATIC MADNESS

ANDREW G. ROBBINS

Bloomington, IN 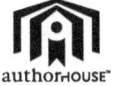 Milton Keynes, UK

authorHOUSE

AuthorHouse™
1663 Liberty Drive, Suite 200
Bloomington, IN 47403
www.authorhouse.com
Phone: 1-800-839-8640

AuthorHouse™ UK Ltd.
500 Avebury Boulevard
Central Milton Keynes, MK9 2BE
www.authorhouse.co.uk
Phone: 08001974150

First published by AuthorHouse   5/5/2006

ISBN: 1-4259-2956-7 (sc)

Printed in the United States of America
Bloomington, Indiana

This book is printed on acid-free paper.

About the Author

Andrew G. Robbins has been a clinical nutritional consultant since 1993. He consults with over 200 chiropractors, medical doctors, pharmacists, naturopaths, nurse practitioners, and osteopaths all over Indiana and Kentucky. Formerly a personal fitness trainer, Mr. Robbins is now a frequent lecturer on nutritional science to many doctor groups in the two-state region, and has been privileged to lecture at many prestigious hospitals and universities, as well as television and radio programs pertaining to health. Mr. Robbins resides in Greenwood, Indiana with his wife, Donna, and their two children, Hannah and Luke.

DEDICATION

To all the brave physicians who have struggled so tirelessly against tremendous opposition and financial difficulty in order to pioneer the coming renaissance in American health care. Each of you is a hero. This book is a small token of my appreciation and admiration.

- Andrew G. Robbins

TABLE OF CONTENTS

INTRODUCTION

What you are about to read may come as a total shock to you.

Since most Americans have been conditioned to revere medical professionals as heroes of our society, your first reaction to the content of this book may be disdainful. You may think me an alarmist, or someone who has a personal vendetta against the medical profession. Whether or not I am an alarmist is perhaps a matter of opinion, but I assure you that I have no personal axe to grind.

The problem with communicating bluntly and forthrightly – as I do throughout this book – instead of taking the reader through a slow and gentle process of paradigm change, is that presenting a case with a barrage of information all at once to a person who holds to a different belief is like trying to wake someone from a deep sleep by dousing them with a bucket of ice water. It is offensive, and because of the reactionary response that often ensues, the argument being presented is not often readily accepted by the hearer (or in this case, the reader). I have found that broaching this subject with some people is almost like trying to convince someone that his lifelong religious convictions are wrong. A person like that will most often not be persuaded in just one or two conversations, especially if the one doing the proselytizing is doing all the talking and simply blasting the hearer with philosophies and facts, giving no opportunity for meaningful interaction. But because I don't have the opportunity to present the facts here in a slow and gentle process, I must ask you to read on with an open mind.

I must also warn you that while I do not go out of my way to be offensive in my phraseology, I also do not attempt to hide my revulsion regarding the issues of which I speak. I believe there are certain issues which call for a strong response; ones that call for people of principle and a strong sense of morality to stand up, casting "political correctness" aside, and declaring that certain things must not be tolerated by our society. That is why I wrote this book.

Yes, I am angry and sickened by much of what is being called, "health care," and I hope you are angry and sickened by what you read here as well – angry enough to do something about it. So because I am a person of principle, I do not apologize for the strong sense of conviction that I convey, and the distinct line I attempt to draw between right and wrong, good and evil.

Lastly, I wish to state that I do not hate conventional medical doctors or any medical professional. In fact, there have been occasions after the writing of the first version of this book that I actually patronized conventional medicine for nagging, minor health issues that my usually-successful nutritional approaches were slow in resolving. Perhaps I was thinking that maybe in the long period of time since I last visited a medical doctor, some things had changed and that maybe someone had gotten "clued in." But the approach to care is always the same, and I inevitably come away from my interactions with conventional medical professionals with the same response and with the same opinion of them.

So while this book may seem like an attack on the medical profession, it is really a declaration to lay people that the caregivers to whom we have trusted our health have misled us – some unknowingly, and some with full knowledge. This book is written, therefore, with the hope that perhaps a few people who have been on a never-ending merry-go-round of conventional medical care may finally be free of their dependence on it and find a more-effective method of healing. It is also written with the hope that maybe there is a minute chance that this book will fall into the hands of a conventionally-trained medical professional whose mind is open enough to reconsider the efficacy of his/her training as the end-all-and-be-all of health care.

To the conventional medical professional who might be reading this, allow me to state that I respect your hard-earned degree. The sacrifices you made to be where you are now are to be commended and appreciated. But let's be open and honest enough with ourselves to put our egos and personal agendas aside, recognizing that growth, progress, and enlightenment often come at the expense of sacred cows, and always requires considering other viewpoints and possibilities.

While I understand that sometimes the bearer of bad news is shot and considered divisive and a rocker of the proverbial boat, it is my hope that somehow this book will serve as my little piece of a larger puzzle that is being pieced together toward the reconciliation of two divided camps, and toward a hopeful future of a united, more effective system of health care.

1

AMERICA'S DEADLIEST THREAT

People are destroyed for lack of knowledge.

-The Holy Bible, Hosea 4:6

The biggest threat to American lives is not terrorism. It is not communism, and it is not war. The deadliest threat to American life lies within our borders. Indeed, there is a stealth, covert enemy among us that has already taken down far more Americans than all of the aforementioned threats combined.

During the Vietnam War era picketers lined the streets of United States cities angrily protesting what seemed to them the senseless loss of American life in the conflict between North and South Vietnam. American government had decided to intervene because communism's growing threat loomed ever stronger, and freedom was at stake for millions of people. But it was not our fight, many argued. And the loss of life, totaling somewhere in the neighborhood of 58,000 American soldiers, was unacceptable to those who opposed our involvement.

Yet, amazingly, a far greater threat has taken far more lives right under our noses here on American soil, but rarely is there a voice raised in protest. And many of the voices that are raised are quickly drowned under the derision of those indoctrinated by the propaganda of our time.

I speak of a plague of cataclysmic proportions. It takes approximately 800,000 American lives every year. It is far worse than AIDS; more insidious than cancer; more catastrophic than the tragedy at the World Trade Center and the Pentagon on September 11, 2001. The plague of which I speak is called, Iatrogenic Disease. What is iatrogenic disease? I'll let the words of William Boyd, M.D., author of the classic medical text, Boyd's Pathology, explain:

> "In fear of the public, we seek refuge in a mystic word, iatrogenic, trusting that the patient will not consult a medical dictionary and find that 'iatros' is Greek for physician, and 'genetic' means caused by. Unfortunately, what is powerful for good may also be potent for evil." (p. 10)

That's right. Iatrogenic disease means sickness caused by the physician. It represents 36% of all hospital admissions and is the nation's leading killer[1], even killing more people than heart disease and cancer.[2] Iatrogenic disease is due to over-prescribing of medications, too many unnecessary and risky surgeries, and simply too much interference with the body's own ability to heal itself by tampering with its biochemistry and chopping up its biomechanics.

In 2000, a presidential task force described medical errors – which is only one source of iatrogenic events – as a "national problem of epidemic proportions." Members estimated that the "cost associated of these errors in lost income, disability, and health care costs is as much as $29 million annually."

For example, in the United States alone, one person dies every 3-5 minutes from causes traceable to side effects of approved pharmaceutical drugs prescribed by the physician, which is almost five times the number of people who die as a result of illicit drugs. Likewise, more people die in the U.S. every year due to medical mistakes than deaths caused by AIDS, breast cancer, or highway accidents, and as many as 9% of all hospitalized patients experience a serious or fatal complication associated with their care.[3] Fourteen percent of cardiac arrests can also be traced to an iatrogenic event.[4]

The Healthcare Symposium Abstracts of Australia stated in 1999 that being a patient in an acute care hospital carries on the average a 200-fold greater risk of dying than being in traffic, and a 2000-fold greater risk than working in the chemical industry.

The Disease Care Industry

There are currently 700,000 medical doctors in the United States. Every year in the U.S. there are approximately 120,000 accidental deaths caused by medical doctors' mistakes.[5] That accounts for 0.171 deaths per medical doctors every year.

Compare those numbers to accidental deaths caused by guns, which is an issue far more protested than medical practices.

There are currently 80 million gun owners in the U.S. Every year there are 1,500 accidental deaths caused by guns.[6] That translates to 0.0000188 accidental deaths per gun owner. In comparison, medical doctors are 9,000 times more likely to kill someone than gun owners! If you factor in the number of people who die from adverse drug reactions every year, the numbers would be staggeringly higher, because at least 106,000 people die every year from adverse drug reactions (ADRs), according to the Journal of the American Medical Association (JAMA). And this number pertains to drugs that were administered correctly. It does not pertain to those that are administered incorrectly, which is not an infrequent occurrence. Likewise, the same study also found that another 2.2 million patients suffer adverse reactions to pharmaceuticals every year, with a majority of those being preventable. [7]

Following is a table showing the staggering figures related to fatal iatrogenic events.

Table 1.

Condition	Annual # of Deaths	Annual Cost	Author
Adverse Drug Reactions	106,000	$12 billion	Lazarou, Suh
Medical Error	120,000	$2 billion	US Dept of Health
Bed Sores	115,000	$55 billion	Xakellis, Barczak
Infections	88,000	$5 billion	Weinstein, MMWR
Malnutrition	108,000	------	Nurses Coalition
Outpatient A DRs	199,000	$77 billion	Starfield, Weingart
Unnecessary Procedures	37,136	$122 billion	HCUP
Surgery Related	32,000	$9 billion	AHRQ
TOTAL:	805,936	$282 billion	

By using Dr. Lucien Leape's 1997 medical and drug error rate of 3 million and multiplying it by the fatality rate of 14%, which Leape used in 1994, we could arrive at an even higher death rate of 420,000 for prescription drug deaths and medical errors combined. If we use these numbers in place of Lazarou's 106,000 prescription drug deaths and the U.S. Department of Health and Human Services' 120,000 medical errors, we could add another 194,000 deaths, making a total of 999,936 deaths annually.

Now let's compare those numbers to the deaths in the Vietnam War. In a nearly ten-year conflict, America lost 58,000 soldiers. That's 5,800 people per year, and there was angry protest in the homeland. BUT CONVENTIONAL MEDICINE KILLS MORE AMERICANS EVERY MONTH (65,328, by conservative estimates) THAN THE ENTIRE NUMBER OF AMERICAN SOLDIERS THAT DIED IN THE TEN-YEAR VIETNAM WAR! So by conservative estimates, nearly 800,000 of our countrymen die every year at the hands of conventional medicine practitioners, and somehow it is mostly accepted without question. In fact, a projected 10-year statistic of 7.8 million iatrogenic deaths is more than all the casualties from wars that America has fought in its entire history.

Why is the morbidity of iatrogenic disease so high? Economic gain appears to be at the root of most of it. In October 1994, the Associated Press published an article entitled, Regulators Wonder if Drugs Prescribed Because of Incentive. The article stated,

> "Drug makers improperly induce doctors and pharmacists to prescribe certain medicines, using marketing incentives that range from direct cash payments to multi-million-dollar research grants, regulators contended. The result can be wrongful treatment (of patients)..."

I have a friend who is a sales representative for a major pharmaceutical company, and he confirmed this report when he confided in me that his company routinely gives away gold-plated golf clubs and Hawaiian vacations to doctors who most frequently prescribe their drugs.

Economic gain also appears to be influencing the doctors in not only how much they prescribe a drug, but how they perform their duties during routine patient office visits. Because the health care system in America rewards numbers, it is to the doctor's economic advantage to get as many patients as possible in and out of the office during the course of a day.

I was in the office of a medical doctor in Louisville, Kentucky a few years ago, and he made a statement that has stuck with me ever since. We were discussing nutritional interventions for Fibromyalgia – a disease pertaining to muscle pain and fatigue. The doctor stopped me in the middle of my dissertation and said, "Mr. Robbins, I'll be honest with you; I'm really interested in nutrition and all that, but I get paid to see patients – I don't get paid to get them well." In other words, he was saying that it would not be in his economic best interest to do a thorough health evaluation on a patient with the intention of treating them with a nutritional approach, because that would take too much time. In the course of time it would take to do a thorough evaluation of one patient, he could see a dozen other patients in the method that he usually practices and make a lot more money doing it.

So in essence, this man's attitude, which appears to be centered around financial gain and not the patient's health, is consistent with that of many of his colleagues. Physicians are rewarded by the system to numbly work their patients through their clinics as if on a conveyer belt, using the same cookie-cutter approach on nearly everyone, which is to ask a question or two, take some vitals (blood pressure and pulse), and then write a prescription or refer out for expensive tests, which he/she often gets a kick-back for. Total time spent with the patient: ten minutes or less. Total fee: astronomical.

The system rewards numbers, not results. So the physician has been conditioned to get the patient in and out as fast as possible with little or no regard for the ultimate outcome. Perhaps that is an unfair blanket statement in lieu of many very caring physicians who do indeed attempt to act in the patient's best interests, but the bottom line largely appears to be economic gain.

In 1995 – before I knew much of what I know now – I was persuaded by an orthopedic surgeon to undergo surgery on my right shoulder to repair torn cartilage in my rotator cuff. The result of the surgery was unfavorable. It devastated my range of motion, and I was worse after the surgery than before. During one of my check-ups I let the surgeon know that I was not happy with the outcome, and wondered if perhaps a mistake had been made. I inquired what could be done to fix my problem without additional cost to me. The doctor became angry at my suggestion, and promptly and rudely ended my office visit. I never saw him again, but went about to pursue legal action against him for restitution of the botched surgery. I soon discovered, however, that laws practically make doctors immune from such actions unless it is a clear case of malpractice. You can take your car back to your mechanic to demand a refund or a re-do of a job that was not completed properly, but you can't sue a medical doctor for mistakes that have been made during "standard procedure." Most tragic of all is that while you can trade in your car if there is a problem that can't be fixed, you can't trade in your health.

Many times the damage done by conventional medicine in permanent and irreversible.

My anecdotal observations aside, statistics overwhelmingly support the assertion that medical doctors are maiming and killing. Nicholas Wade of Science Magazine reported, "Every year a million people – 2% to 3% of all hospital admissions – are admitted primarily because of a negative reaction to drugs." (Science Magazine #179)

It has also been reputed that 5% of all hospital patients contract new infections AFTER they have been admitted, affecting 2 million people annually and accounting for as many as 80,000 deaths. For those who survive, hospital acquired infections increase hospital stays an average of seven days, and subsequently increase medical bills enormously.[8,9]

I can personally attest to the occurrences of these hospital-borne infections. A year or so after I had written the first edition of this book, one of my beloved uncles underwent gallbladder surgery – a relatively simple procedure, as surgeries go. Shortly thereafter he began complaining of pain and sickness. His physician assured him there was nothing to be concerned about, and did not examine him to discover the source of the discomfort. Five days after the surgery, my uncle was dead from a staph infection he had acquired while in the hospital.

Modern medicine is also responsible for 7,000 deaths per year due to errors in administering medication,[10] 12,000 deaths per year from unnecessary surgeries,[11] and 20,000 deaths per year due to other various mistakes made in hospitals.[12] But nowhere is the iatrogenic character of modern medicine better revealed than during doctor strikes.

When MD's went on a fifty-two day strike in Bogata, Colombia in 1976, for instance, there was a subsequent reduction in the death rate of 35% during that time, according to the National Catholic Reporter. Also in 1976, doctors in Los Angeles went on strike to protest malpractice rates in Los Angeles County, and the death rate dropped 18% as a result. In Israel, there was a doctor's strike in 1973 that lasted one month. The Jerusalem Burial Society reported that the Israeli death rate dropped FIFTY PERCENT that month! The last time there had been such a dramatic reduction in the death rate was twenty years before, the last time the doctors had been on strike.

Even those who work alongside doctors know the risks involved in being under their care. One group of 10,000 nurses was questioned about hospital preferences, and a third of them said they would refuse admissions to the very hospitals in which they worked. Even more alarming was that more than 40% of the nurses said they had witnessed doctors make errors that resulted in the patient's death.

It is statistics such as these that moved Dr. Robert Mendelsohn, M.D., author of the brave books, Confessions of a Medical Heretic, and, How to Raise a Healthy Child in Spite of Your Doctor, to state:

> "I believe that more than 90% of modern medicine could disappear from the earth – doctor, hospital, drugs, and equipment – and the effect on our health would be immediate and beneficial." (Confessions of a Medical Heretic, from the Non Credo)

Ivan Illich, likewise, was compelled to conclude:

"Among all our contemporary experts, physicians are those trained to the highest level of specialized incompetence." (p. XIV Medical Nemesis)

To qualify, I want to state emphatically that I am not against having medical doctors as an integral and important part of our medical system. I would not have my two wonderful children and my lovely wife to help raise them if it weren't for the skills of talented medical doctors that performed C-sections when my wife was in distress and unable to deliver our babies through her birth canal. I am thankful for our superior emergency medical technology. As far as health care goes, however, conventional medicine is not the answer, as we can plainly see. In fact, the term "health care" is really a mislabeling. Conventional medicine is really disease care or crisis care. Crisis care seeks to control or manage disease by manipulating body systems through invasive drugs and surgery rather than to support the body's own ability to heal itself. Crisis care seeks to ease symptoms but, in most cases of chronic disease, does not address the origin of the problem. Crisis care excels in addressing acute trauma and injuries, but it falls short in supporting optimal health. If you want true health care or preventive care, don't go to a conventional medical doctor. If I had a broken bone that needed to be set, or an inflamed appendix that needed to be removed before rupturing; or if I was in a terrible accident and had internal bleeding; or if I needed sutures in a deep gash, a medical doctor would be the best qualified to meet those needs. But if I had heart disease, cancer, osteoporosis, diabetes, Irritable

Bowel Syndrome, arthritis, back or neck pain, depression, Chronic Fatigue Syndrome, Fibromyalgia, high cholesterol, high blood pressure, or some other chronic disorder, a conventional medical doctor is the last kind of physician whose care I would seek.

It is clear from the evidence that modern medicine hasn't the faintest notion how to effectively ward off the scourges of our culture. Heart disease is the second-leading killer of Americans, taking 669,697 American lives annually[13], and cancer isn't far behind at 553,251 annual deaths.[14] There are currently 18.2 million people in the U.S. who have diabetes, and an estimated 5.2 million more already have it but have not yet been diagnosed. There are currently 3,500 new diabetes diagnoses made every day.[15]

Modern medicine does not have a magic pill or a wonder surgery that has made even a minute difference in those statistics. In fact, the British Medical Journal in 2000 published epidemiological findings indicating that at best only 15% of allopathic medicine has a good scientific basis. So as much as 85% of conventional medical interventions are based on conjecture and unproven ideas, and you are the unwitting guinea pig.

It is no small wonder, therefore, that modern medicine does not have the answer to our society's ills. But there is one thing that modern medicine has been very good at doing, and that is duping the American consumer into believing that their methods of treatment are based on sound research while every other healing art that competes with them are not.

In Dr. C. Evert Koop's Surgeon General Report of 1989, he reported that 7 out of 10 Americans die due to "lifestyle diseases," which are chronic diseases like heart disease, cancer, diabetes, etc, that are preventable. Rarely, however, do we hear from the medical community regarding how to effectively prevent these plagues. In fact, it would seem from outward appearances that it is in the medical community's economic interests to keep the public somewhat ignorant about healthy living, because disease care is big business. Each balloon angioplasty procedure, for example, which is performed to try and open up clogged arteries, costs in excess of $14,000 per operation, and there are more than 300,000 of them performed each year. But because of the short term benefits of that procedure (studies show that arteries close up again in 57% percent of all balloon angioplasty patients), and because a 1992 study published in the Journal of the American Medical Association found that half of all the angioplasty surgeries carried out in the U.S. were probably unnecessary, The American College of Cardiologists was compelled to ask, "Is angioplasty being done for cardiologists or for patients?"

But, of course, the more aggressive alternate surgery for cleaning out blocked arteries is bypass surgery at the tune of $43,000 per procedure.

Drug therapy, likewise, is enormously profitable for both the doctors and the pharmaceutical industry. Why else do you think they are now using television commercials to get you interested in Lipitor and Clarinex and all the others? And while doctors and drug companies are growing ever richer, the American public is being raped by insurance companies and growing still sicker in spite of all the high-tech medical interventions.

Indeed, America has the finest emergency medical system in the world, and our diagnostic capabilities are breaking new ground as well with the development of tools like CAT scans and others. Our technical wizardry is now being turned to even more dramatic interventions like artificial hearts, transplantation of vital organs like the heart, kidneys, and liver, and microsurgeries that provide the capability to reattach severed limbs. Likewise, high-tech medicine is now being turned toward the bizarre by providing sex change operations; and the vain, by providing facelifts and other cosmetic surgeries.

As wonderful as some of the aforementioned advancements are, one would expect our culture to be healthier and living longer as a result. But is that the outcome of high tech medicine? Hardly. In fact, the increases in life expectancy that have occurred since the first part of the 1900's have been attributed in large part to improvement in hygiene. While better hygiene habits have been successful in helping to control infectious disease, chronic degenerative diseases continue to proliferate and ravage our culture. In his book, Medical Nemesis, Ivan Illich wrote:

> "After a century of Utopia, and contrary to current conventional wisdom, medical services have not been important in producing the changes in life expectancy that have occurred..."
> (p. 5)

One study showed that America ranked 12th among 13 industrialized nations comparing measurements of health in the general populations.[16] Think of it! The wealthiest and most technologically advanced nation on the planet has not been able to produce a healthy society.

Following is a list of America's health statistics.

- Only 1.5% of our population is considered optimally healthy[17]

- Cardiovascular disease affects 64 million Americans and represents 38.5% of all deaths.[18]

- One in seven women get breast cancer at some point in their lifetimes.[19]

- Forty nine percent of all Americans suffer from at least one chronic disease, and one of every five children under the age of seventeen has already developed some chronic disorder.[20]

- Cancer kills more than a half a million Americans every year.[19] Cancer is the number one non-accidental cause of death in children.[22]

- Nearly 43 million American adults are afflicted with arthritis (20.8%).[21]

- More than 70 million people (1 in 4) suffer some form of serious digestive disorder.[23, 24]

- Twenty-five million Americans are migraine sufferers, and migraines have increased 50% in the last 20 years.[25]

- Cardiovascular disease, cancer, and diabetes alone account for nearly 2 of every 3 deaths in the U.S.[26]

In spite of our technological advancements, it appears that America is indeed the land of the free, but the home of the diseased. We're swallowing more pills, submitting to more injections, being sold more and more surgeries, and coughing up more money than ever before, but we have virtually nothing to show for it. Even after spending 1.6 trillion dollars each year on health care, Americans are not as healthy as many nations whose health care budgets are a fraction of ours. So what gives?

2

The Medical Juggernaut versus the New Health Care Paradigm

The doctor of the future will give no medicine, but will interest his patients in diet, exercise, and care of the human frame.

-Thomas Edison

The original motives for the development of the Western healthcare system by early Americans were probably more noble than they have presently become, but there was always an underlying philosophy regarding healthcare that lacked the same insight that was demonstrated when our Founding Fathers forged the Declaration of Independence and the Constitution. Most mainstream physicians in early America believed that the traditions of Europe were not hearty enough to flourish in the vigorous New World. Benjamin Rush, for example, who was a signer of the Declaration of Independence and himself a medical doctor, stated that American doctors should beware of placing "undue reliance upon the healing powers of nature in curing disease."[27] Apparently influenced by the philosophies of the Enlightenment and the mentality of the frontier, Americans have always embraced new ideas and technologies as "better," and believed that it was always advantageous to do more rather than less. Aggressive bloodletting and strong purging, for example, were standard therapy for many diseases in the early years of the Union. In fact, it is thought that bloodletting may have been the ultimate cause of the death of George Washington. Medical professionals in general were less interested in valid science than in quick results and would engage patients in an ongoing process of experimentation by trial-and-error. They often prescribed copious amounts of tonics and stimulants of questionable medicinal efficacy, sometimes consisting of mind-altering substances like opium.

While the motives of many of the country family doctors who made house calls may have been caring and noble, it was actually early in our history when the elitist attitude among medical doctors first began. It mattered not that many of the healing methods of Europe and Asia were working, and even many of those by Native American Indians, for that matter. What mattered was that Americans were "enlightened," and American medical professionals appeared to want to distance themselves from all other "lesser" systems of healthcare. This, of course, eventually led to all manner of excesses in American medicine, and the excesses of the nineteenth century stimulated the growth of various alternative therapies based upon hygiene, nutrition, and herbal and folk remedies. Chiropractic and osteopathy originated in the Midwest during this era, and homeopathy, likewise, was transplanted into the United States after having first been developed in Germany.

All the different alternative sects of healing differed among themselves significantly in their methods, yet they all shared the traditional philosophy that diseases are not distinct entities to be specifically treated as such, but rather are manifestations of disharmony and imbalance within the systems of the body. As these alternative sects grew in prominence, their influence and popularity was noticed by the conventional medical establishment. In 1897, the dean of medicine at Tulane University, in fact, complained that "quacks [are] the greatest foe to the medical profession... [an] obstacle to the financial success of the reputable medical practitioner."[28]

Yes, it has always been about money and power. The medical profession has been consistently and relentlessly hostile to alternative methods of healing.

Chiropractic, for example, has always been the arch enemy of the medical establishment because of its effectiveness and popularity. In 1962, the general counsel of the Iowa Medical Society, Robert B. Throckmorton, devised a plan to "contain" chiropractic in the state by encouraging "ethical" complaints against chiropractors and opposing the coverage of chiropractic services by health insurance, worker's compensation, and labor unions. The following year, the American Medical Association invited Throckmorton to implement chiropractic containment nationwide, and its board of trustees voted to establish a Committee on Chiropractic (the name of the committee was later changed to the Committee on Quackery) that considered its "prime mission to be, first, the containment" and "ultimately the elimination of chiropractic."

In 1966, the AMA House of Delegates adopted a resolution to ensure that medical doctors understood that they were forbidden to associate with chiropractors. The Judicial Council ruled that a physician would be guilty of unethical conduct if he or she even lectured to a group of chiropractors on a health-related subject. One member of the Committee on Quackery stated at a workshop of the Michigan State Medical society that a medical doctor would be acting unethically if he or she referred a patient to a chiropractor for any reason whatsoever.

In 1976, Chester Wilk and four other fellow chiropractors filed an antitrust suit against the AMA and seven other medical associations and four individuals, alleging a conspiracy to eliminate chiropractic through refusal to associate professionally with chiropractic physicians. Eleven years later in 1987, the AMA and its codefendants were found guilty of boycott and conspiracy, and a permanent injunction was issued preventing the AMA from restricting association with chiropractors. The AMA lost a subsequent appeal in 1990.[29]

While the court decisions prevented the AMA from restricting medical doctors from professionally associating with chiropractors, the enmity between the two groups reverberates to this very day. While the walls seem to be slowly coming down with certain individuals, the medical profession as a whole still reviles and alienates chiropractors for the most part, and do not consider them to be "real" doctors.

Ask any medical doctor what he/she thinks of chiropractic medicine, for example, and most would respond with a sharp jab at chiropractic physicians, indicating that they are not really doctors at all. "They go to school for two years and come out calling themselves doctors," I have heard some say. The truth, however, is that chiropractors are required to have no less than eight years of schooling, and all of them have significantly more hours of education in anatomy, physiology, and diagnosis, which means that chiropractors probably know more about how the body works than most MDs, and are more highly trained in how to spot dysfunction. The few areas that medical doctors are trained more highly in are specific to conventional medicine, such as pharmacology (the administration of drugs), surgical procedures, etc. [30] (see table 2).

Table 2

Class Description	Student Hours =	Chiropractic	Medical
Anatomy		520	508
Physiology		420	326
Pathology		271	335
Chemistry		300	325
Bacteriology		114	130
Diagnosis		370	374
Neurology		320	112
X-Ray		217	148
Psychiatry		65	144
Obstetrics & Gynecology		65	198
Orthopedics		225	156
TOTAL HOURS		**2,887**	**2,756**
Specialty Courses		1,598	1,492
ENTIRE TOTAL HOURS		**4,485**	**4,248**

While most medical doctors seem to conveniently forget that research indicates that chiropractic care is more beneficial that drugs and surgery for a number of different health concerns such as back pain, colic, menstrual cramps, high blood pressure, bed-wetting, to name just a few [31,32,33,34,35], it is also true that no one has ever died at the hands of a chiropractor like is so common in the medical profession.

The ongoing bias against chiropractors is demonstrated in the fact that in many states they are not allowed to perform certain medical procedures that they have been sufficiently trained in, such as performing breast exams or drawing blood.

A chiropractor friend of mine in Indianapolis, Indiana, for example, told me that he had a female patient several years ago who came to see him in tears. When he inquired what was wrong, she explained that her right breast was persistently tender and she feared the worst. But her medical doctor assured her nothing was wrong and sent her on her way. When she pressed the issue later, again her doctor persisted in his assurance that nothing was the matter. So now she was in the office of my friend, asking him to do a thorough breast exam. My friend explained that although he was indeed trained in doing breast exams, by state law he was not allowed to perform any since he was a chiropractor. But the patient would not take no for an answer. She was in obvious distress, and trusted her chiropractor enough to all but force him to do the exam. With him still insisting he could not do the exam, she disrobed above the waist and begged him to proceed. Reluctantly, he performed the exam, and found that she indeed had a tumor. He explained to the patient that he could not diagnose cancer under state law, but strongly suggested that she go above the head of her medical doctor and schedule an appointment with an oncologist that very day.

Sure enough, the patient came back to my friend's office some time later in tears again, but this time they were tears of thanksgiving. She explained how the oncologist's findings were positive for cancer, but that they had caught it in the very early stages, and because of the early detection the chances were very good that she would survive. She credited her chiropractor with saving her life.

Chiropractors are not alone, however, in their persecution at the hands of the medical establishment. Homeopathic physicians are all but extinct in this country because of the movement to eliminate them. According to medical historian Harris Coulter, the 1846 formation of the American Medical Association was a direct response to the founding of the American Institute of Homeopathy two years earlier.

The AMA maintained a hostile position toward homeopathy throughout the remainder of the 19th Century, and between 1850 and 1880, medical doctors were sanctioned for even associating with homeopaths. A New York physician was expelled from his medical society in the late 1870's, for instance, for purchasing milk sugar – which was used in preparing homeopathic preparations – at a homeopathic pharmacy. So staunch was the opposition toward homeopaths that one medical doctor in Norwalk, Connecticut was punished when he came under suspicion of having consulted with a homeopath, who happened to be his own wife! [36]

The unceasing persecution toward homeopaths by the medical community took a heavy toll, and by the 1930's homeopathy was on the brink of extinction in the United States.

Even as recently as the early 1970's, a medical dictionary defined homeopathy as a "cult" and stated that its only real value "was to demonstrate the healing powers of nature and the therapeutic virtue of placebo."[37]

The obvious bias by the medical establishment against any other healing method that competes with them is demonstrated in the fact that they refuse to acknowledge that any of the alternative healing arts have value when it is clear from reams of research that chiropractic, homeopathy, naturopathy, and herbal and nutritional medicine (to name just a few) are extremely efficacious. This bias exists in spite of the fact that research also suggests that conventional medical methods do not have any real power to heal the body in the case of chronic disease, but simply address symptoms.

In spite of this evidence that medical doctors are, as Ivan Illich said, trained to a high level of specialized incompetence, I never cease to marvel at their pomp. To the average medical doctor in America, medicine is almighty, and any healing art that ventures off the path of what is considered conventional is lambasted as "quackery."

In America, conventional medicine seems content to stick with what obviously doesn't work, while vilifying and ridiculing the competition. In many European countries, however, drugs and surgery are considered last resorts, and it is the alternative health care methods in America that are considered mainstream there. In fact, only 10 to 30% of people worldwide use what America considers "conventional" medicine, and 70 to 90% use alternative medicine regularly.[38] Chiropractic, naturopathy, homeopathy, herbal medicine, nutritional therapies, etc, are commonplace in healing institutions all across Europe and Asia, and they have the health to show for it.

Likewise, there is now a heretical movement away from invasive medicine to more natural means by which to treat dysfunction and maintain health among some medical doctors in the U.S. who are disillusioned with conventional medicine and who have more concern about their patients' health than they do their income. I call this movement away from the conventional medical model heretical because many of these brave physicians are ostracized by their colleagues and labeled as heretics. Many must give up a substantial percentage of their previous income in order to practice according to their convictions, and still others are harassed by their state licensing boards.

One such doctor who endured untold suffering at the hands of the state licensing board was Dr. Walt Stoll, formerly of Lexington, Kentucky. Dr. Stoll was a conventionally trained medical doctor who eventually became very ill. Dr. Stoll soon realized that the very medicine he had practiced for many years could not cure him of his chronic ailments, so he began educating himself on natural medicine. Having completely cured himself in a few short months using natural methods, Dr. Stoll resolved to begin helping his patients in the same way. He founded an integrated medical clinic near Lexington in Nicholasville, Kentucky that offered chiropractic, herbal and nutritional medicine, and a host of other natural as well as conventional medicine. Dr. Stoll's clinic soon became known internationally, and he drew patients from all fifty states and several foreign countries.

Sadly, Dr. Stoll's disillusionment with conventional medicine soon turned to disdain as the Kentucky State Licensing Board constantly harassed him with charges that threatened to strip him of his medical license if he did not discontinue his unconventional methods of treatment. He fought them for years at his own expense. Finally, the Board trumped up a list of false charges against him and revoked his license. Financially depleted and weary of fighting, Dr. Stoll retired from practice and moved to Panama City, Florida. He has since authored an excellent book entitled, Saving Yourself from the Disease Care Crisis.

This attempt by the people in power to squelch anything that threatens their places of prominence is nothing new. It has been a common theme down through history. But perhaps more disgusting than this initial attempt to squelch life-saving information is that when it seems apparent that the proliferation of information cannot be contained or covered up, the opponents will do a one-eighty and loudly proclaim the benefits of a "new discovery," giving themselves credit for having discovered it. I predict that within a few short years of this writing, the money-mongers in power in conventional medicine will attempt to lobby to allow medical doctors and physical therapists to do chiropractic adjustments, and if successful, they will then issue a proclamation of the benefits of chiropractic manipulation; only, they will not call it "chiropractic." They will use a term like "spinal therapy" or something similar in order to obscure the real origin that was born over 100 years ago.

In addition to the growing interest and success of chiropractic medicine, other healing arts are also becoming more commonplace in America. Nutritional medicine, in particular, is enjoying unprecedented success and growth as more people are educating themselves regarding the benefits of various vitamins and herbs, and as more doctors are experimenting with nutritional interventions as alternatives to drugs and surgery.

In fact, in 2002 the Journal of the American Medical Association (JAMA) released an article reversing the AMA's longstanding policy regarding doctors recommending supplements to their patients. It is now the position of the AMA that doctors should recommend to all their patients, especially the chronically ill, that they at least take a multiple/vitamin mineral supplement daily.[39] (I have since heard from a medical doctor that the pharmaceutical companies have threatened to stop advertising in their journal if the AMA continued to publish articles about the benefits of nutrition, and in response to the prospect of losing all that advertising money, JAMA has since reverted back to minimizing the benefits of dietary supplements.)

In November of 1995 JAMA released an article entitled, Learning How Phytochemicals Help Fight Disease, in which they stated that "phytochemicals [the nutritional constituents of plants] are important in the prevention and treatment of malignant disease."[40] The article cited several studies in which researchers were able to reverse malignancy in laboratory animals using high doses of phytochemicals. In fact, the article quoted Dr. Pamela Crowell, PhD, at Indiana University School of Medicine, who stated that she conducted a study to determine how many oranges one would have to eat everyday in order to get a therapeutic level of limonene (which is present in only the pealing). The answer was 400! In other words, it is impossible for a cancer patient to get enough of the nutrients known to help the body fight off malignancy simply by altering the diet alone. The conclusion of the JAMA article was that supplementation with phytochemicals is a must for cancer patients, and is strongly recommended for everyone, especially for those who do not eat at least five servings per day of fresh fruits and vegetables.

Another compelling study on the benefits of chromium and grape-seed extract supplementation on subjects with Syndrome X and advancing age stated, "...the current paper will encourage people to seek a better lifestyle and use of appropriate dietary supplements, which may favorably affect life-span and reduce incidence of advancing age-induced chronic disorders and improve deleterious symptoms of Syndrome X."[41]

These "therapeutic lifestyle changes" are considered first line therapy by some circles of medicine, and are recommended by the National Institutes of Health, Centers for Disease Control and Prevention, American Heart Association, Arthritis Foundation, North American Menopause Society, American Association of Endocrinologists, National Institutes on Aging, and many others.

So replete is the research pertaining to the benefits of supplements and therapeutic lifestyle changes in the scientific literature that it is feasible that it may one day be considered medical malpractice (or at least medically irresponsible) for doctors to fail to recommend these to their patients. And if that day ever does come, America will be a healthier society because of it. It is these interventions, after all, that have been among the primary treatments of choice by conventional doctors in Europe and Asia for generations. So then, if the information pertaining to the benefits of supplements and lifestyle changes is so replete in the scientific literature, why aren't more medical doctors recommending them? That's an excellent question, and one that we will examine in more detail in the next chapter.

3

A CORRUPT ALLIANCE

"...Many powerful individuals within the organized medical profession...are aware of this information [regarding serious and fatal reactions to drugs], but appear to have an implicit agreement to obscure the facts, minimize the truth, and deceive the public."

-Neil Z. Miller, from *Vaccines: Are They Really Safe and Effective?*

It seem curious why empires like the pharmaceutical industry and the American Medical Association would appear to fail so miserably in promoting healing methods that would truly benefit the patient instead of simply prescribing more drugs. Aren't these organizations devoted to improving health? Yes, it would appear that health and vitality are the motives, but appearances can be deceiving.

The drug companies, as well as the American Medical Association, have done their part in the suppression of life-saving information in an effort to protect their financial interests. They have already been pressuring the FDA to regulate the nutritional supplement industry in the hopes that vitamins and herbs will be considered "drugs" and will only be available through medical doctors. In doing so, the money-hoarding drug companies will strip all other supplement manufacturers of their ability to distribute food supplements to the general public and will have monopolized the industry. Legislation of this nature has already been attempted, and if it wasn't for the watchful eye of good men like Senator Orin Hatch of Utah, these bills would have already been passed into law. If bills like this ever do pass through into law, you can bet that drug companies and medical doctors will suddenly change their tune and begin announcing from the highest rooftop the benefits of taking vitamins.

The FDA exemplifies how Washington bureaucracy can corrupt otherwise reasonable ideas in the pursuit of power and profit. The FDA was originally established to protect public health, but many of the actions by the FDA have instead threatened it – primarily because the agency has entered into a corrupt alliance with the very pharmaceutical industry that it is supposed to be regulating. This has resulted in the FDA allowing harmful medicines to reach the public, costing hundreds of thousands of lives and untold human suffering. Yet, unthinkably, the agency has acted to block safer alternatives like certain nutritional supplements and other natural methods of treatment, because those alternatives threaten the pharmaceutical industry's chokehold on healthcare.

The Journal of the American Medical Association published an article in May of 2002 that illustrates just how big the problem has become. The article pertained to a study reviewing the history of all drugs approved by the FDA between 1978 and 1999, and it found that over 10% of the total number of drugs approved were later found to have potentially lethal side effects or were withdrawn from the market as unsafe. When the researchers narrowed their analysis to the most recent drugs approved by the FDA, the figure rose to 20%.[42] This means that there is now a 1 in 5 chance that a drug approved by the FDA is lethal!

One reason this is the case is because of conflicts of interest within the FDA. For a drug to be approved, it must first be reviewed by an unbiased advisory committee. After reviewing the clinical data on the drug's safety and efficacy, the committee then votes on whether or not to approve it. However, a review of the official records of 159 advisory committee meetings held between January 1, 1998 and June 30, 2000 revealed that in 55% of the meetings that took place during that time period, at least half of the participants had a financial conflict of interest. An incredible 92% of the meetings had at least one committee member with a conflict of interest! In other words, many of the very committee members that were reviewing the data for a drug's approval either had stock in the company's drug that they were reviewing, or had some other similar conflict of interest that would make it financially advantageous for the committee member to approve the drug! It is not too much of a stretch to imagine, likewise, that many of the drugs that do not reach the public are denied approval because of the same financial conflicts of interest.

But this is not the only financial conflict of interest going on between the FDA and the pharmaceutical industry.

In 1992, there was a debate between the pharmaceutical industry and the FDA regarding how fast drugs were being approved. The pharmaceutical industry complained about the long delays in new drug approvals, and the FDA claimed that it lacked the financial resources to speed up the process. So in that year, Congress passed the Prescription Drug User Fee Act (PDUFA) in response to the debate, which is a program that enables the FDA to charge a fee for new drug applications that they would then use to hire additional staff. But it isn't too difficult to see how the user fee program is becoming the tail that wags the dog, because it is now the drug industry that is footing the bill for FDA staff to review and approve new drugs.

In a recent budget request, the FDA called for user fees to increase to $295 million. This equals roughly 17% of the administration's total budget. The fees would add 500 FDA positions funded by the drug industry, bringing the total number of FDA employees funded by the pharmaceutical industry to 1,530, which translates to approximately 1 in 7. More importantly, the new positions mean that 55% of all committee members reviewing new drug approvals would now be paid by the pharmaceutical industry! "The fox would essentially be in charge of the chicken coop," observed columnist Kathleen Dole.

Dole likewise noted, "What may be the most pernicious aspect of the alliance between the FDA and the industry it is intended to regulate is the incentive it creates to stifle the growing competition from alternative and complementary medicine. "

One must understand that this incentive is motivated out of a desire to maintain power and control in the healthcare industry – even if it means suppressing potentially life-saving information – and nutritional medicine represents perhaps the biggest financial threat to the fortress of conventional healthcare. In fact, polls indicate that 69% of Americans use some form of unconventional medicine,[43] and the sales of dietary supplements have experienced yearly double digit growth.[44] But in spite of this clear demonstration of the public will, Congress has had to act on two separate occasions to assure that the public would still be able to purchase these products.

In 1966, the FDA attempted to classify nutritional supplements as drugs if the products had potencies greater than 150% of the Recommended Dietary Allowance (RDA). Keep in mind that the RDA's are the bare minimum the body requires for function. The RDA for vitamin C, for example, is barely enough to prevent the tissue disease, Scurvy. So classification of this nature was clearly not a health issue, but a financial one. After a decade of controversy, a significant public uprising, and a huge legislative battle, Congress finally passed the "Proxmire Amendment" that blocked the FDA action.

The FDA, however, has not given up easily, because despite the Proxmire Amendment, it will periodically attempt to extend its regulatory power to include supplements. Finally in 1994, in apparent exasperation with the FDA, Congress passed the Dietary Supplement Health and Education Act (DSHEA) with the intention of preventing the FDA from unduly limiting consumer access to food supplements. The DSHEA enabled supplement manufacturers to make health claims about their products as long as it was accompanied by "significant scientific agreement." However, in an apparent attempt to manipulate the DSHEA for its own benefit and the benefit of its allies in the drug industry, the FDA interpreted the phrase, "significant scientific agreement" to mean the supplements had to pass the same clinical trial process as prescription drugs at a cost of hundreds of millions of dollars. Moreover, it excluded from consideration studies pertaining to the safety and efficacy of supplements by other federal agencies such as the NIH and the CDC. In other words, it didn't matter if supplements were beneficial or not. All that mattered was whether or not the FDA said they were, and they refused to admit that any supplement had any benefit.

In response to the FDA's ludicrous pronouncement, two enraged supplement distributors, Sandy Shaw and Dirk

Pearson, went to court over it. In a landmark decision, the U.S. Court of Appeals for the District of Columbia instructed the FDA to allow supplement manufacturers to make true statements about their products. Can you grasp the significance of that? A federal court had to force the FDA to allow people to tell the truth!

If this weren't enough, the FDA also issued 568 "warning letters" between 1997 and 2000 to pharmaceutical companies for offenses ranging from false and misleading advertising to substandard manufacturing practices. It seems obvious, however, that what they called warning letters were simply attempts to make themselves look unbiased, because in nearly every case, no penalty was imposed for the violations. Conversely, supplement manufacturers are rarely warned; they are simply shut down or at least forced to stop selling certain substances – even when there is a question as to whether or not the offense actually occurred.

For example, the entire supplement industry was forced to stop selling the amino acid, L-tryptophan, when a few people died in the early nineties who were taking it in supplement form. It was never established why the individuals died. Was it a manufacturing issue, or is there something toxic about tryptophan? Common sense tells us that the former had to be the case, because millions of people ingest tryptophan in food form all the time when they eat turkey or they drink green tea. Yet the government never bothered to examine this issue thoroughly, but simply decided to ban all tryptophan supplements.

Why then doesn't the government ban Ibuprofen – to use just one example of many – since 16,500 deaths per year occur as a direct result of the gastrointestinal complications brought on by Non-Steroidal Anti-Inflammatory (NSAIDs) drugs? This double standard is shocking, but it is inspired by the people in power in an attempt to crush any competition which threatens their financial fortresses.

More recently the Federal Trade Commission brought legal action against the world's largest professional supplement company, Metagenics, for claims made about its bone product, Cal Apatite. Metagenics decided to fight the charges rather than to acquiesce, like other entities in similar situations are forced to do because of the financial burden created by the long legal battles. The outcome was positive for Metagenics and the supplement industry at large, because after reviewing all the evidence pertaining to the efficacy of the product, the judge ruled largely in favor of Metagenics. But the company spent one million dollars defending itself – an amount not easily absorbed by a company in an industry that is miniscule compared to the size and financial power of the drug companies.

Even more shocking is that when the distributor of a natural sweetener called Stevia attempted to sell cookbooks instructing consumers how to use the product, the FDA promptly ordered him to destroy them, dispatching agents to his warehouse to supervise their burning. It is interesting to note that one of the officials in the FDA at one time had financial interest in NutraSweet, with which Stevia directly competes.

Dr. Jonathan Wright, M.D., a noted expert in the field of alternative and nutritional medicine, had his office raided by a SWAT team when FDA officials solicited help of King County, Washington police to confiscate "dangerous drugs." Only later did they discover what they were confiscating was actually injectable vitamins!

These kinds of extreme actions are being taken despite the fact that of the 140 million Americans who say they take food supplements regularly, only 2,500 adverse events are even remotely related to food supplements each year, with death being almost never. Yet 2.2 million people have dangerous reactions to their prescription drugs every year, and 106,000 die.

The 2002 conclusion of the Women's Health Initiative Study, which revealed that hormone-replacement drugs can cause heart disease, stroke, and cancer, and do not help prevent bone loss as was originally advertised, is a perfect example of how criminally irresponsible the drug company and the FDA have been. Why weren't these facts known BEFORE the drugs were released to the public? Why wasn't the research done by the FDA and the drug companies before millions of women – 38 percent of postmenopausal women in the U.S., in fact – were exposed to these dangerous drugs? Why were six million women unwitting guinea pigs for drugs that had insufficient testing prior to their approval by the FDA?

In 2004, a South Carolina medical doctor, Jim Shortt, who practices integrated medicine, was falsely accused of killing a female Multiple Sclerosis patient, supposedly by applying a hydrogen peroxide IV to get rid of viruses and bacteria. Armed Federal, State, and local law enforcement agents, in an almost "Waco" style assault team, complete with body armor and assault weapons, stormed his clinic and seized everything in sight.

Although medical literature clearly shows that hydrogen peroxide IV therapy has been around for almost 100 years with over a million treatments performed with NO DEATHS ever recorded, the mere allegation of death by this method, false as it was, and made by an elected politician with no medical training, caused a massive assault by US law enforcement.

In 2004 a popular joint pain medication was recalled amidst headlines that it caused heart attacks and strokes. Why wasn't this dangerous drug prevented from coming to market in the first place? Why were millions of Americans exposed to this potentially fatal drug? The fact is, prescription drugs undergo rigorous trials costing millions of dollars prior to their release in order to identify possible side effects. Therefore, it is reasonable to assume that the pharmaceutical giant who made this arthritis drug knew about these risks prior to its release, but they released it anyway. Why? Could it be that the executives apparently believed that any future possibility of lawsuits was worth the risk in lieu of the billions of dollars to be made in the short run? It apparently didn't matter to the executives at this particular drug company that tens of thousands of people were going to develop chronic cardiovascular disease taking their drug. The FDA now reports that 55,000 people were killed using this COX-2 inhibiting drug.

Columnist Arriana Huffington wrote an article published in the New York Times, November 24th, 2004, called, You Want a Moral Issue? How About Drugs that Don't Kill?, in which she stated regarding the killing of the 55,000 people who took this arthritis drug at their doctors' recommendation, "there ought to be a special place in hell for corporations that show such a wanton disregard for human life." I couldn't agree more.

It is simply unfathomable to me that so many Americans are raising cries of outrage over our involvement in Iraq while largely remaining silent over corporations that are killing thousands of Americans and lining their pockets with unequalled wealth while they do it. Most Americans have apparently been subtly brainwashed that this is acceptable.

In a just world, the executives of the various drug companies and the committee members in the FDA would be charged with criminal recklessness and manslaughter for the countless numbers of people who have died unnecessarily because of being prescribed drugs that should never have been on the market in the first place. We learned from the Enron scandal that we must hold industry leaders personally responsible for their actions, and that criminal indictments are absolutely necessary. Some of the executives at Enron got what they deserved, but I don't expect that to happen any time soon with the executives of Merck or any other pharmaceutical company, because these drug lords are helping to fund the FDA – the very organization that is supposed to be regulating them. So when public health is sacrificed on the altars of the great gods of money and power, nearly anything goes, and there is rarely retribution for the guilty.

4

Your Response

The old "take a pill and make it better" mentality is the biggest health problem we face in our society today. We think that as long as we can take a pill that stops our nose from running, we're healthy; that if gulping down laxatives keeps us regular, we're improving the condition of our body. But, if we are ever to achieve and maintain true health, we have to understand what health really is. We need to stop thinking in terms of treating illnesses, and start thinking in terms of creating wellness.

> -Dr. Terry Rondenberg, DC,
> from *Under the Influence of Modern Medicine*

THE BOTTOM LINE

The bottom line is that the pharmaceutical companies – and the doctors who they sell their drugs to – are motivated by money. These doctors are rewarded by insurance companies for the numbers of people they see – NOT how good they are at getting people well.

Conversely, ancient China's medical system seems odd on the surface, but it served to motivate the doctors to keep people well. Each household in China was required to pay a monthly fee to their family physician, and if someone in the household became ill, the payments stopped until health was restored to that individual. This way, it was in the physician's best interest to keep the members of each household on his list vital and healthy.

In America, however, long gone are the days of doctors who make house calls and who are sincerely more concerned with your health than they are making the payment on their winter house in the Caribbean. Long gone are the days when insurance companies exist to make sure you get good health care no matter what.

The fact is, we have devolved into a nation of opportunists that worship money. This appears to be true at the highest levels of government and business, right down to the next door neighbor.

This degeneration of our moral compass is perhaps demonstrated best in our health care system. A health care system is supposed to exist to help people, not harm and rob them. While this was no doubt the incentive when our healthcare system was first in its developmental stages, it has now devolved into a system that has largely eclipsed the patient.

In his stellar book, The Four Pillars of Healing, Dr. Leo Galland, MD, stated regarding the lost focus of getting people well by our healthcare sytem,

> The eclipse of the patient…is the most profound, lasting, and unfortunate effect of [modernized medicine]: its insidious and destructive success in altering relationship between physicians and patients. For the doctor in training, the patient was to become an object of study, stripped of personal identity, plucked from the context of life and placed in a hospital bed. Here, the

process of diagnoses and treatment would be increasingly directed by the wonders of technology..." (pg. 22).

The American medical system in its present state cannot exist for too much longer. If it continues to operate in its present state, where doctors are rewarded for keeping patients sick and insurance companies deny treatment of inexpensive natural methods but willingly pay for all monstrously expensive drugs and surgery, it will eventually bankrupt itself. One way to force a change before something catastrophic happens is to vote with your dollars. Do not rely on conventional medicine for your general health care needs. For general care, find a good naturopath or chiropractor, or even an MD who practices integrated medicine. And by all means, take responsibility for your own health by eating sensibly, exercising, and augmenting the diet with high-quality nutritional supplements.

Since 1990, there have been more visits to alternative practitioners in the U.S. than conventional ones,[45] so the tide is beginning to turn. In fact, a number of studies indicate that the more education a person has, the less likely he/she is to trust or use the services of traditional allopathic physicians. But it is the American Medical Association and the drug companies who still have a chokehold on healthcare because of their power and financial resources. Therefore, they still have an immense ability to control the information you see and hear. Who do you think sponsors all those drug commercials you see on prime time television every evening, and the impressive full color glossy ads you see in magazines? And because drug companies are now a major source of advertising dollars for networks and magazines, there is also a financial interest in reporting news by these major media outlets that shows pharmaceutical drugs in a positive light, and puts anything that competes with this juggernaut in a negative light.

One would need to look no further than the 2004 report apparently showing that vitamin E increases the chance of heart attacks and stroke. Well, guess who partly funded that study. A drug company! So why would a pharmaceutical company want to help fund a study on something natural? Could it be that they knew the outcome of the study before the study was even conducted? In other words, it only stands to reason that a drug company would want to help fund a study on a vitamin E only if they knew ahead of time that the outcome of the study was going to show that ingesting vitamin E was not beneficial to human health, thus diminishing the public's interest in the competition of nutritional supplementation. In fact, the Council of Responsible Nutrition (CRN) rebutted the vitamin E study by saying that its methods did not meet the standards of true scientific scrutiny and the conclusions were absolutely wrong.[46]

It is obvious that we cannot trust the drug companies and the medical community at large to provide us with information that is going to benefit us. It also seems apparent that these various medical and government entities are more motivated by money than they are people's health. So by denying conventional doctors your patronage, sooner or later they must be forced to face the truth if enough people rely on other healing methods by which to maintain their health.

EDUCATED PEOPLE CHOOSE ALTERNATIVE HEALTH CARE

Studies show that people who choose natural methods of healing tend to be more educated than those who rely on conventional medicine alone. An article in the Annals of Internal Medicine reported a study in which researchers from the University of Pennsylvania Cancer Center compared the education level of 304 of their Center's own medical patients and 356 patients who sought natural healing therapies that conventional medical doctors consider " unorthodox," "unproven," "ineffective," "fraudulent," and so on. Table 3 demonstrates that people who chose natural methods of healing tended to be substantially more educated on the average.

Table 3.

People who choose natural alternatives to traditional medicine tend to be significantly more educated than those who rely on medicine alone.

Level of Education	Chose Medicine	Chose Alternatives
High School graduate or less	62%	40%
Attended some college	18%	24%
Bachelor's degree	9%	16%
Graduate degree	11%	19%

When researchers asked why the more educated people leaned so heavily toward methods of care that conventional medicine considers "quackery," they found that these individuals were attempting to cure their cancer by "strengthening their own adaptive powers," and conventional medicine doesn't give them that choice. In the words of the researchers, the alternative methods of treatment "are geared toward improving the patients' own biological and psychic capacity to counteract illness." (The term "psychic," when used to describe the patients' capacity to counteract illness, was not meant to describe some mystic experience or power. It simply means that each individual has built within us by our Creator an ability – both physical and mental – to combat illness.)

In stark contrast, the California Medical Association (CMA) describes people who prefer non-medical therapies as "unsuspecting," "gullible," "desperate," and "alienated" victims of health fraud. Dr. Dean Black, PhD, in his excellent book, Health at the Crossroads, stated,

> "Anti-quackery advocates use the term 'health fraud' to describe all therapies that conventional medicine doesn't approve of, with virtually no standard of discrimination." (pg. 93)

Indeed, former president of the National Council Against Health Fraud, Inc, Dr. William T. Jarvis, Ph.D., lumped herbalists and health food therapists in with witches and faith healers. He rhetorically presented the view of orthodox medicine when he asked:

> "Should we license and give Medicare dollars to alchemists, witches, herbalists, health food therapists, faith healers, etc., on the assumption that the consumer will be wise enough to choose the proper kind of care, and within sufficient

time to protect his life and health?"

Dr. Jarvis obviously doubted the wisdom of consumers and lay people to choose for ourselves.

Dr. Dean Black points out:

"Physicians may not doubt our wisdom when they meet us as friends, but when they accept us as patients, and particularly when they reach into their arsenal of tests and therapies, their training virtually requires that they see us as helpless and needing to be controlled. Choosing external control as a strategy, and deciding that people ought to be controlled, are two sides of the same coin. And notice how each principle assumes about consumers exactly what it assumes about the body. The medical principle assumes that neither the body nor the consumer is wise; the natural healing principle assumes they both are, or at least they are capable of becoming so." (From Health at the Crossroads, page 92)

In an article appearing in USA Today, FDA Deputy Commission John Norris defined health fraud, in essence, as anything performed outside of an approved clinical setting by anyone who is not a licensed medical doctor. In reading the CMA booklet and all other anti-quackery literature, you could reasonably substitute the phrase, "people who choose non-medical therapies," for the phrase, "victims of health fraud." The CMA booklet explains why "gullible," "alienated," "unsuspecting," and "desperate" people become "victims of health fraud."

> "Chronic diseases tend to be viewed by these persons not as separate disease entities, but rather as external symptoms of an internal underlying dysfunction, disorder, or toxicity and, therefore, these patients are susceptible toward treatments geared toward improving their overall wellness, and strengthening their own biological and psychic capacity to counteract illness."

Actually, the phrase, "treatments geared toward improving overall wellness, and strengthening their own biological and psychic capacity to counteract illness" precisely describes natural healing principles. According to conventional medicine, however, improving wellness and strengthening one's own capacity to counteract illness is apparently a bad thing. They would evidently prefer that we be chronically ill so that we can rely on "approved" methods of care – their care.

EMPOWERING YOURSELF

The Information Age is a wonderful time to be alive. At the click of a button on our "mouses" we can access reams of information on nearly any subject. Also, retail book outlets like Borders and Barnes & Nobles provide a smorgasbord of materials on hundreds of subjects. Likewise, many of today's health food stores typically have book shelves with excellent reading on health-related topics.

One must be cautious, however, of believing everything you hear and read. There are opportunistic charlatans in every industry and walk of life, and natural healing is no exception. There are duplicitous supplement companies, dishonest chiropractors, and greedy "integrative care" medical doctors. So let the buyer beware.

Typically, however, even the opportunistic alternative health care practitioners will usually do a fairly good job of addressing the health needs of their patients. Some of them may simply want to lock you into long-term care way beyond what is reasonable, give you sacks full of supplements, or inappropriately charge your insurance company.

For chiropractic care, I recommend that you seek out someone who practices in a "diversified" style, since there is no one-size-fits-all approach to chiropractic care. Likewise, do not allow a chiropractor to talk you into a long-term contract of two or three times a week care for months and months. Any honest chiropractor will tell you that most conditions that present themselves can be resolved in just a few weeks of regular care (2-4 visits per week), and any subsequent maintenance care can be once a month or so.

Regarding supplementation, there may be some doctors who want to talk you into taking basketsful of vitamins. While aggressive vitamin therapy may be indicated for a brief period of time (a few weeks or months, depending on the condition), it is never appropriate, in the view of most nutritional medicine doctors, for a patient to take dozens of supplements at a time. The body will only absorb so much in any given dose. Furthermore, I would not recommend purchasing your supplements from a grocery store or retail chain store, by internet or mail-order, or from a multi-level company. Most of the nutritional companies who sell to these entities do not perform the appropriate quality control measures to ensure a high-quality, efficacious product. It is my recommendation to purchase your supplements from a doctor who practices nutritional medicine and who uses a professional doctor's line of nutritional supplements.

While it is important to beware of charlatans, in my experience these types of practitioners are few and far between. Most chiropractors, naturopaths, and clinical nutrition specialists are not in their line of work to make a lot of money. If money was their focus, they would have become conventional medical doctors. Most of these "alternative" practitioners are not making huge amounts of money doing what they do. Like Dr. Walt Stoll mentioned earlier in the book, most of these caring practitioners gave up the prospect of making a lot of money so that they could practice health care according to their convictions.

Optimally, it is best to live a lifestyle that provides you with the best opportunity to avoid having to go to a doctor at all, and rely on one of the alternative healing methods when you do need care. Educating yourself is paramount in learning how to care for yourself and your family so that a doctor won't have to. While this book is not dedicated to providing that kind of information, I can recommend a few resources to help you get started and arm yourself.

- The book, *Prescription for Nutritional Healing*, by Dr. James Balch, MD, and Phyllis Balch, C.N.C. (Avery Publishing), is a very popular resource as a reference guide for ways to treat many common ailments nutritionally. Many health food stores carry this book.

- One of my other books, *Achieving Physical Excellence and Vitality*, is an instruction guide in choosing healthy foods, choosing the best and most appropriate supplements, and how to get the most out of exercise. It reviews a fair amount of research pertaining to all of these areas. The primary focus of this book is to provide a guide by which to achieve dramatic results in losing weight and accomplishing radical physical transformation in a short period of time. It is available on my website, www.shofarpublications.org.

- Dr. Ben Lerner's book, *Body By God*, is very popular and is a very complete guide in how to overhaul and tune up one's health. It covers exercise, diet, stress management, and other issues pertinent to one's well-being. It is published by Thomas Nelson Publishers.

- *Body for Life*, by Bill Phillips, is a great motivational book for achieving greater fitness and rejuvenating one's health. In addition to some very helpful instructions regarding diet and exercise, Phillips also includes the stories and before/after photographs of several individuals who have made radical physical transformations in a short period of time using his methods. Phillips' book is published by Harper Collins.

- *Eat, Drink, and Be Healthy*, by Dr. Walter C. Willett, M.D., is another option for those wishing to inform themselves on how to eat healthier, as the book is devoted exclusively to the subject of better health through better eating.

- *The Four Pillars of Healing*, by Dr. Leo Galland, is a highly acclaimed book among alternative medicine practitioners. It not only provides insightful and well-documented insight on how to achieve healing naturally, but it also looks at the medical establishment from the perspective of the author, who is himself a medical doctor. Dr. Galland's book is published by Random House.

- Dr. Adriane Fugh-Berman, M.D., has authored a book entitled, *Alternative Medicine: What Works*, that I feel is an honest and very comprehensive look at a number of healing arts. Her book is published by Odonian Press.

- The book I mentioned earlier, *Saving Yourself from the Disease Care Crisis*, by Dr. Walt Stoll, tells the story of conventional medicine through the eyes of a licensed physician who has experienced both sides. Dr. Stoll also devotes much of his book as a how-to in preventing and treating many of today's common ailments with lifestyle modification, diet, and nutrition. His book is available online at Amazon Books, or by calling the publisher at 1-800-464-7034.

- *Under the Influence of Modern Medicine*, by Dr. Terry A. Rondenburg, is a very comprehensive look at the destructive influence of Western Medicine. It is published by The Chiropractic Journal.

- Dr. Janson's *New Vitamin Revolution* is a revision of Dr. Michael Janson's first highly-acclaimed book, The Vitamin Revolution. It is probably one of the most complete books you will ever find pertaining to the research on and use of dietary supplements.

- *Fast Food Nation: The Dark Side of the All-American Meal*, by Eric Schlosser, is a meticulously researched account of how the fast food industry is transforming not only our health as a culture, but also our landscape, economy, workforce, and society.

- *Beating the Food Giants,* by Paul A. Stitt, takes an inside look at the food industry and how food manufacturers are radically changing the nutritional value of food for the sake of profit. Paul Stitt is formerly a biochemist with the Quaker food company. His book is published by Natural Press.

- *Sugar Blues,* by William Dufty, is still as timely and profound today as when it was first published in 1975. It is 234 pages of absolutely jaw-dropping information on the poisonous effects of sugar. It is published by Warner Books.

- *Super Size Me* is a documentary movie about a man who performed his own experiment on the health consequences of eating fast food by consuming nothing but McDonald's for 30 days. It is fascinating and very informative. Wal-Mart carries copies, and you can rent it in most video stores.

- A great movie on the politics of insurance and health care is *John Q,* with Denzel Washington. It is a Hollywood drama, but paints a fairly accurate portrayal of how the bureaucracy of insurance and health care have eclipsed the needs of the patient.

Other than educating yourself, another response is to keep the pressure on your legislators to take actions that will protect your rights, and to let your voice be heard on issues pertaining to public health. One way to do this is to call or write your congressman and senators. Writing or calling your Senators and Congressman has great impact since not many people do it. They need to hear from you regarding these issues. In addition, it is important to stay abreast of what is happening in the arena of legislation since the FDA on several occasions has attempted to widen their circle of power by attempting to push through laws that would regulate the supplement industry, as I described in the previous chapter.

5

The Road Less Traveled

Someone once said that one definition of insanity is doing the same thing over and over while expecting different results. Some people expect to lose weight, to have more energy, to get over their chronic health problems, or simply to feel more vital, but they never do anything to bring about the changes they are hoping for. They continue to consume the same junk food day after day, they continue to live inactive lives, they continue to live under chronic stress, and they may continue to indulge other bad habits such as smoking or drinking too much alcohol. Even if they do make a few minor changes, many people do not stick with those changes long enough to make them a lifestyle so that it results in a dramatic impact on their health. So a year passes and their health does not improve. Then two years; then five; then ten. And before they know it, their health has degenerated past the point of no return.

The same seems to be true of the kind of health care people tend to seek out. Because they have been conditioned so successfully all their lives by the conventional medical model, they may read something like this book and get motivated for awhile, and decide to patronize health care alternatives the next time they need care. But the enthusiasm sometimes wanes after they sit through hours of television programming that consists of dozens of drug advertisements. So when the day comes that they need care, it is so easy to fall right back into what is familiar.

That is the way of human nature. We are creatures of habit. So allow me to warn you that making the changes necessary for vital health and longevity will take forethought, planning, and energy. You won't wake up tomorrow morning and all the sudden be Mr. Fitness or Mrs. Health Food Mom just because you got temporarily motivated by something you read. Significant physical improvements will take education and then application, both of which take time and hard work. Likewise, you may not sense a strong attraction to visit an alternative health care practitioner the next time you need care. Your tendency will perhaps be to do what is easy and familiar.

These are times when you must dig deep into the strength of your character in order to carry out your good resolutions. Cavett Robert said, "Character is the ability to carry out a good resolution long after the excitement of the moment has passed."

Allow me to also warn you that your good resolutions will not be welcome changes by many of your friends and family members. You might be labeled as a "health fanatic," and laughed at as an extremist. Sometimes your commitment to healthy eating may be very uncomfortable for the people with whom you dine. There have been occasions when people have said to me that they feel "guilty" when they eat certain foods in my presence, for example. While I am not advocating shoving your convictions down others' proverbial throats, it is now apparent to me that the very strength of one's resolve and the ability to carry it out in social situations shines a spotlight on the bad habits of others, and sometimes makes them uncomfortable.

They may feel that you think less of them because of their choices.

I recommend doing your best to make people feel at ease and let them know that it doesn't bother you for them to eat any way they want, but that you have made a resolution and you are doing your best to stick to it.

One way to defuse any future ridicule that you might endure at the hands of friends, family, and co-workers, is to give out copies of this book and allow them to see for themselves the truths you have come to embrace. Help them to see the difference between crisis care and wellness care, and encourage them to patronize the physicians who are providing wellness care unless they have a crisis. (By the way, you can usually find these physicians under Holistic Physicians in your yellow pages.)

Sharing profound statements like the following quote from Emory University Health Sciences Center regarding the benefits of lifestyle changes can sometimes make a difference with people who are open:

> "Many patients with classic cardiovascular disease risk factors can achieve risk reduction goals without medications within only three months of initiating therapeutic lifestyle changes."[47]

Even presenting profound evidence such as the quote above sometimes will not persuade those who are too proud to acknowledge their ignorance, or who defend their lifestyles because they know that they lack the willpower and/or the desire to change. It is true that people tend to take the road of least resistance. Ordinary people tend to adhere to the status quo. However, extraordinary people who accomplish the extraordinary never take the road of least resistance. Hamilton Mabie said, "Don't be afraid of opposition. Remember, a kite rises against – not with – the wind." Booker T. Washington said, "You measure the size of the accomplishment by the obstacles you had to overcome to reach your goal."

Indeed, we have seen from much of the information that we have covered already what the status quo has done for the health of the average American. Status quo living often results in fatigue, disability, obesity, degeneration, and disease. I hope it is now firmly established in your mind that lifestyle is THE MAJOR factor in disease, and even in less severe forms of ill-health. Medical science has now conclusively shown that most chronic diseases are ones of lifestyle, and that lifestyle changes can result in significantly better health.

A study in the New England Journal of Medicine showed, in fact, that 91% of diabetes cases, for example, are attributable to lifestyle habits and forms of behavior that differed from those individuals who were at low risk.[48] In other words, people who were at low risk to diabetes had good lifestyle habits. People who were at high risk had poor lifestyle habits.

Furthermore, another New England Journal of Medicine study stated,

> "Not only do persons with better health habits survive longer, but in such persons, disability is postponed and compressed into fewer years at the end of life."[49]

From time to time someone will joke with me that "we all have to die of something; you might as well go out enjoying yourself," or "you can eat right and exercise all your life and then die anyway." But in America, most people who live well into their "Golden Years" do so with a significant degree of degeneration and disability. For these, the Golden Years are not so golden. So perhaps going out of this life enjoying yourself by indulging all that your appetite craves and then eventually giving your ailing body over to conventional medicine for them to experiment on is a fine way to live as long as you don't mind growing old having to wear a diaper because you can't control your bowels, or not being able to remember who your children are, or needing a staff girl at a convalescent center to feed you mashed potatoes while you drool on yourself, or having to wear a catheter because you no longer have a bladder, or taking a half a dozen medications for all your ills, and another half dozen to offset the side effects of the first six, etc. But that's not how I want to go out of this life. I want to go out like Dr. Linus Pauling.

Dr. Linus Pauling won the Pulitzer Prize for his groundbreaking research on vitamin C. Dr. Pauling was a staunch advocate of healthy lifestyle habits combined with nutritional supplements. He lived well into his nineties, and was still physically active and intellectually keen until his death. He experienced very little, if any, disability and degeneration. Without much warning, Dr. Pauling simply laid down and died one day.

Scripture provides some fascinating and profound insight here regarding lifestyle and self-control. Proverbs 23:1-3 says,

When you sit to dine with a ruler, note well what is set before you, and put a knife to your throat if you are given to gluttony. Do not crave his delicacies, for that food is deceptive.

This passage of the Holy Bible was written approximately 4,000 years ago, and is attributed to the great Israelite monarch, King Solomon. In that time and place, it was only the rulers, dignitaries, and wealthy who ate rich foods on a regular basis, consisting of lots of animal fat and refined carbohydrates. The commoners subsisted on fresh fruits, vegetables, grains, and wild game. While the commoners experienced very little degenerative disease, these scourges were commonplace among the rich. Heart disease, cancer, arthritis, and other chronic degenerative diseases were so common among the cultural elite that they were called "the diseases of kings and queens."

In modern America, nearly everyone – rich and poor alike – eats like the wealthy dignitaries of the ancient Middle East. (Actually, we eat worse than that, since even ancient dignitaries did not consume the incredible amount of chemical food additives that modern Americans do.) Therefore, we have an entire nation of people who are plagued with the diseases of kings and queens.

Regarding verse 3 of Proverbs 23 – *Do not crave his delicacies, for that food is deceptive* – it is an interesting study to consider what is meant by "deceptive food." In the context of this passage, it is reasonable to conclude that deceptive food could refer to any food that looks good, smells good, and tastes good, but is not good for you. That pretty much describes 80-90% of everything Americans stuff into their mouths. So when our bad habits catch up with us, the most common mentality is to get a prescription or undergo surgery in order to cover over the symptoms brought on by the bad habit so that they are no longer noticeable, and then we can go on indulging our bad habits without a care – that is, until the next physical malfunction. So making the necessary changes that will ultimately result in greater health and vitality will require a complete paradigm shift. That paradigm shift will completely cut against the grain of what we as a culture have come to accept as normal.

Every person who has ever accomplished anything notable – whether it was physical, spiritual, financial, or whatever the goal – did it on a road less traveled by their peers. They often did it alone. They often did it while enduring ridicule and/or alienation. But the fact that they did not let detractors pull them off course is why they now stand out among their contemporaries. Whether the individual is famous or not, every person who has ever accomplished anything notable each have one thing in common, and that is their resolve to go against the crowd and pursue their convictions and passions.

That is the theme of Robert Frost's famous poem, *The Road Not Taken*.

> "...Two roads diverged in a wood
>
> And I took the one less traveled by
>
> And that has made all the difference."

I sincerely hope that this book has been eye-opening for you. Even more I hope that this information will not simply be interesting trivia, but that it becomes useful in compelling you to action. It is, after all, knowledge resulting in action – not just the knowledge itself – that leads to positive changes.

May God bless you in your pursuit of greater health.

References

1. Dean C, Feldman M, Null G, Rasio D, *Death by Medicine*, Nutrition Institute of America, 2003-2004, www.nutritioninstituteofamerica.org.

2. *National Vital Statistics Reports*. Vol. 51, No. 5, March 14, 2003.

3. Brennan, T.A. et al, *Incidence of Adverse Events and Negligence in Hospitalized Patients*, The New England Journal of Medicine 324(6); Feb 7, 1991: 370-376.

4. Dubois, R.W. and Brook, R.H., *Preventable Deaths: Who, How Often, and Why, Annals of Internal Medicine* 109: Oct. 1, 1988:582-589.

5. U.S. Dept of Health and Human Services.

6. U.S. Bureau of Alcholol, Tobacco, and Firearms.

7. Lazarou J, Pomeranz BH, Corey PN. *Incidence of Adverse Drug Reactions in Hospitalized Patients: A Meta-Analysis of Prospective Studies*. JAMA 1998 Apr 15;279(15). 1200-5.

8. *National Nosocomial Infections Surveillance (NNIS) Systems: National Nosocomial Infections Surveillance System Report, data summary from October 1986-April 1998,* issued June 1998. Am J Infect Control 1198 Oct;26(5): 522-33.

9. *Center for Disease Control.* Public Health Focus: Surveillance, Prevention, and Control of Nosocomial Infections. MMWR 1192; 41:783-7.

10. Phillips DP, Christenfeld N, Glynn LM. *Increase in US Medication-Error Death Between 1983 and 1993.* Lancet 1998, Feb 28;351(9103):643-4.

11. Leape LL. *Unnecessary Surgery.* Anna Rev Public Health 1992; 13:363-83.

12. Lazarou J, Pomeranz BH, Corey PN. *Incidence of Adverse Drug Reactions in Hospitalized Patients: A Meta-Analysis of Prospective Studies.* JAMA 1998 Apr 15; 279(15): 1200-5.

13. *National Vital Statistics Report.* Vol. 51, No. 5, March 14, 2003.

14. IBID.

15. American Diabetes Association, www.diabetes.org/ diabetes-statistics.jsp.

16. Starfield B. (2000, July 26). *Is the U.S. Health Really the Best in the World?* Journal of the American Medical Association, 284(4), 483-485.

17. U.S. Department of Commerce and the Bureau of the Census, Statistical Abstract of the United States, 1992.

18. American Heart Association, 2001. www. americanheart.org/presenter.jhtiml?identifier=4478.

19. The National Cancer Institute's (NCI) Surveillance, Epidemiology, and End Results (SEER) Program. SEER Cancer Statistics Review 1975-2001.

20. U.S. Department of Commerce and the Bureau of the Census, Statistical Abstract of the United States, 1992.

21. Summary Health Statistics for U.S. Adults, 2002.

22. Summary Health Statistics for U.S. Children, 2002, Table 10.

23. Horwitz BJ, Fisher RS. *The Irritable Bowel Syndrome*. New Engl J Med, 2001;344:1846-50.

24. Mayer EA. *Emerging Disease Model for Functional Gastrointestinal Disorders.* Am J Med 1999; 107(5A):12S-19S.

25. National Headache Foundation, 1999.

26. ACS/ADA/AHA *Scientific Statement, Preventing Cancer, Cardiovascular Disease, and Diabetes,* Circulation. 2004;109:3244-55.

27. Quoted in W.A. Silverman, "Doing More Good than Harm," in *Doing More Good than Harm: The Evaluation of Health Care Interventions: Annals of the New York Academy of Medicine*, Vol. 703 (1993), p. 5.

28. S.E. Chaille, *The Practice of Medicine as a Money-Making Occupation,* New Orleans Medical and Surgical Journal, Vol. 49 (1897), p. 608.

29. Moore, JS. *Chiropractic in America.* John Hopkins University Press, 1993, Baltimore MD: 131-37.

30. Based on a review of curriculum catalogues from eleven chiropractic colleges and twenty-two medical schools in the United States.

31. Moore, JS. *Chiropractic in America.* John Hopkins University Press, 1993, Baltimore MD:16.

32. Klougart N, Nilsson N, Jacobson J. *Infantile Colic Treated by Chiropractors: A Prospective Study of 316 Cases.* Journal of Manipulative and Physiological Therapeutics 1989;12(4):281-88.

33. Kokjohn K, Schmid DM, Triano JJ, Brennan PC. *The Effects of Spinal Manipulation on Pain and Prostaglandin Levels in Women with Primary Dysmenorrhea.* Journal of Manipulative and Physiological Therapeutics 1992; 15(5):279-85.

34. Morgan JP, Dickey JL, Hunt HH, Hudgins PM. *A Controlled Trial of Spinal Manipulation in the Management of Hypertension.* Journal of the American Osteopathic Association 1985; 85:308-13.

35. Reed WR, Beavers S, Reddy SK, Kern G. *Chiropractic Management of Primary Nocturnal Enuresis.* Journal of Manipulative and Physiological Therapeutics 1994; 17:596-600.

36. Starr P. *The Social Transformation of American Medicine.* Basic Books, Inc/Harper, 1982, New York:98.

37. *Stedman's Medical Dictionary,* Williams and Wilkins, 1972, Baltimore MD:583.

38. NIH. *Alternative Medicine: Expanding Medical Horizons* (U.S. Government Printing Office, 1993), liv.

39. Fletcher, RH, Fairfield, KM, *Vitamins for Chronic Disease Prevention in Adults,* JAMA, June 19, 2002. Vol. 287, No.23.

40. Marwick C. *Learning How Phytochemicals Help Fight Disease.* JAMA. Nov. 1, 1995;274:1328-1330.

41. Preuss HG, Debasis B, Bagchi M, *Protective Effects of a Novel Niacin-Bound Chromium Complex and a Grape Seed Proanthocyanidin Extract on Advancing Age and Various Aspects of Syndrome X.* Ann NY Acad Sci 2002;957:250-59.

42. Temple RJ, Himmel MH, *Safety of Newly Approved Drugs: Implications for Prescribing.* JAMA 2002 May 1, Vol 287 No. 17, p. 2273.

43. Haskell; Stanford University National Survey, September 1998.

44. O'Donnel, J. *Neither Food Nor Drug: Dietary Supplements Fall in Regulatory, Medical Gray Area.* USA Today; June 19, 1997.

45. Eisenberg DM, Kessler RC, Foster C, et al. *Unconventional Medicine in the United States: Prevalence, Costs, and Patterns of Use.* New England Journal of Medicine 1993; 328:246-52.

46. Council for Responsible Nutrition (CRN), *CRN Questions Conclusions Reached by Researchers in Recent Vitamin E Meta-Analysis.* Nov. 2004. Retrieved online at www.crnusa.org.

47. From the Emory University Health Sciences Center. American College of Cardiology, 53rd Scientific Session – March 9, 2004.

48. Hu FB, Manson JE, Stampfer MJ, Colditz G, Liu S, Solomon CG, Willett W, Diet, *Lifestyle, and the Risk of Type 2 Diabetes Mellitus in Women,* N Engl J Med 2001;345(11):790-97.

49. Anthony VJ, Richard TB, Hubert HB, Fries JF, *Aging, Health Risks, and Cumulative Disability,* N Engl J Med 1998;338:1035-41.